Will Thou Be Made Whole

Hope and Healing through Nutrition and the WORD

A special thanks to my friend Tammy for the idea to help others by sharing my story and my wonderful husband James for his support and editing skills.

by Cheryl McGuire

All Scripture quotations are taken from the _Holy and Authorized King James Bible_

Cheryl McGuire's Facebook Page: Will Thou Be Made Whole
Email: bemadewhole23@gmail.com

Preface

Hope and healing: in sharing my story I want to give you hope.

Hope: that there is more to life than sickness and disease. Hope and healing: because there is a wonderful God who loves and cares for you and designed you for so much more.

Healing: because too many people are hurting with both physical or emotional pain. While food may aide your body to heal physically, God is the Great Physician who can heal us from the pain of abuse or neglect.

Whatever your pain, the answers can all be found in the Word.

In this book, I give God all the credit for my healing and He has the right to tell me "No, I AM enough" at any time as I continue this journey.   I am a work in progress with my peace and joy coming from the Lord. He has further blessed me by placing me in a country and a time where Bibles can be openly found and can be freely studied. This is not the case for many parts of the world, and too many take it for granted. Count yourself blessed if you are able to study openly and freely the Word of God.

I should not be here today; in fact, 2014 is the year I should have died. God, however, had other plans……. so this journey began.

But they that wait upon the LORD shall renew [their] strength; they shall mount up with wings as eagles; they shall run, and not be weary; [and] they shall walk, and not faint. Isaiah 40:31

Fear thou not; for I [am] with thee: be not dismayed; for I [am] thy God: I will strengthen thee; yea, I will help thee; yea, I will uphold thee with the right hand of my righteousness. Isaiah 41:10

Now faith is the substance of things hoped for, the evidence of things not seen. Hebrews 11:1

Table of Contents

This book is designed as a companion guide for a healthy, whole food lifestyle where you eat food as close to the way God made it as possible.

Disclaimer

The information contained in this book is based upon my personal journey; the results may not be typical. Your results will vary based upon your unique medical history and DNA. I am not a medical professional. This book is for educational and informational purposes only: it may not be construed as medical advice. Any medical information provided is, at best, of a general nature. It cannot substitute for the advice of a medical professional. Any information provided contained within is subject to change. You are encouraged to confirm any information obtained from or through this book with other sources. I encourage you to seek medical advice before starting any new program regarding any medical conditions or treatment needs.

My Journey

God has been guiding this journey from the beginning, I give Him the glory for the improvements in my health, and for all His guidance, in the form of putting people in my path at the right time who had the next piece of the puzzle. I cannot wait to see the finished, whole person I am meant to be.

Why "Will thou be made whole?" you may wonder. About a year into this journey (and during a book study to be discussed later), I heard a message at church on John 5:1-15. As many times as I had read or heard this story it never occured to me that Jesus was asking a question. Did he want to be made whole? You think he would have answered Jesus with a loud "YES." Instead, he made excuses. It resonated with me: I was the one standing there being asked, did I want to be made whole. At this time, I had to fight for every pound lost, for every health gain, and it was tough. I was eating well, but still struggled with cravings and being hungry all the time. But He was there, He was willing and able to show me the correct path. All I had to do was be open to learning. I have healed mentally, physically, and spiritually. I hope this book helps you do the same.

May 2014 . . . I was dangerously sick and could not stop gaining weight, no matter how closely I followed the medical nutritionists' diet while also taking diet pills. I could do very little except go to work, then come home and rest . . . so I could go back to work the next day. I had to take breaks when I got up from my desk, and planned my trips to get as much done in as few steps as possible. I kept getting more diagnoses, but no answers as to why I kept getting autoimmune illnesses, (full list to be discussed later). The only answers I got were, "This is how we manage this illness;" "It's only going to get worse;" and "The only hope is to slow the progression." Also, I had non-alcoholic fatty liver disease, and would soon need gallbladder removal surgery. My asthma was so bad that I could not walk very far without taking a rest break and using a rescue inhaler. I was letting my housework go, doing only the minimum each day. I was scaring my husband and children with my wheezing and lack of energy.   I was falling apart and aging prematurely. The turning point was when I asked my church for prayer for a non-surgical way to heal my gallbladder. HIS ANSWER . . .

The first piece of the puzzle was found on a flyer at the gas station. A new chiropractor (Dr. Mel - Dr. Melanie Gartside) was opening a Maximized Living office. The flyer said that if you were dealing with a number of health issues, they could help. Almost all of my diseases were listed. I was skeptical, and did some research on them (read lots of review, both the good and bad) . . . but I was desperate for help, so I took a chance. I showed up even as they opened the doors at their grand opening celebration and set up my first appointment.

Their approach was different than the chiropractor I had previously seen. It included getting my spine back to its correct position, along with targeted supplements, and nutrition. The nutritional approach was the exact opposite of what the MD's office had me eating. It stressed real, whole foods, and cutting out grains and sugar wherever possible and adding in healthy fats. And it worked.

I had found out that I was gluten intolerant about a week before coming to Dr. Mel's and the medical doctor had just noted it in my chart, but had no advice for me. Nothing. I was overwhelmed. But the Maximized Living diet plan was already gluten free, and Dr. Mel was willing and available to answer my questions. As it turns out, I was also malnourished: yes, at a size 28/30 I was malnourished! But in fixing it this, my health started improving. I was getting off of medications, but only lost about 15 pounds over 18 months. I had stopped counting calories, stopped gaining weight, while eating real food. What an amazing difference only a few weeks made! Then Dr. Mel started offering educational classes that discussed various topics that I needed. All I had to do was be ready to hear and put them into practice.

2nd piece of the puzzle - One of above classes had a guest speaker, a doctor who specialized in cases like mine. I made an appointment and joined her program. I found out I had a leaky gut and a large number of food sensitivities. She did a very complete panel of blood tests, and used targeted supplements. She had me further change my diet to eliminate the food sensitivities, and also avoid nightshades for a while (such as peppers, tomatoes or potatoes) to give my gut a chance to heal. She also changed my thyroid medicine to a compounded medicine, so I quit having low thyroid symptoms. No weight loss, but again my health continued to improve.

3rd piece of the puzzle came in the form of a book study: <u>A Course in Weight Loss: 21 Spiritual Lessons for Surrendering Your Weight Forever</u> by Marianne Williamson. Over the years, I had tried every diet out there: I would only lose a few pounds and gain back more, while hungry all the time. In the course of this book study I discovered many things about myself that I did not even realize were holding me back. Growing up, I had been the victim of physical and emotional abuse. But I also had some really great mentors. Turns out I had a lot of issues around food, and being forced on diets as a kid. At that time I did not have any weight to lose, and would have health issues when I lost a few pounds. As an adult, I would punish myself with food, and used the excuse of being stressed or using weight as a protective layer. I felt that I did not deserve to be a healthy weight, so when I would start to lose weight, some part of me would panic, the weight loss would stop and I would gain it back. Until I did this book study I did not even realize that I was doing this. Having learned it, I now had a choice. I could continue as I had in the past, or I could change and move forward.

I learned that talking about your issues only makes your brain relive what happened, but in writing out the information you are able to let things go and heal. Another benefit of writing, for me, was once I got started, my subconscious would bring up random issues to be dealt with. This book study was emotionally tough, but it was one of the most rewarding things I have done: to release all of the mental reasons I held onto the weight. I have found peace with the abuse of my childhood, but not necessarily with my abusers. God is still working on that one.

4th piece of the puzzle - Therapeutic massage: I won a door prize for a free massage. I started getting regular massages and they were helping my muscles to relax. This allowed my spine and ribs to move more freely into place at the chiropractor's. Psalm 139:13-16 began coming alive.   She would hit a sore spot and was able to follow signals to where the actual knot started. Often that spot was nowhere near the area that hurt, but my body was compensating for it. It helped my overall health and mobility.

5th piece of the puzzle - Naturopathic doctors: who were able to use my body to test and guide me to herb blends that worked with my body to heal itself. The muscle testing was more accurate than the blood work that the MD ran. The great thing was no side effects.   Again, real, whole food nutrition was stressed.

6th piece of the puzzle - Online summits: thanks to the Internet we are now able to attend health summits in the comforts of our own homes. Years ago, you would go to a convention center and listen to expert after expert give their lectures. I have learned so much about nutrition, and our body's ability to heal through listening to some of the world's best functional medicine specialists. The one thing most had in common was that they all started with their own health issues, and in learning to help themselves, they became better healers. Often they had changed their specialty, or even switched to another medical model to better help their patients.

The first one I heard was "The Fat Summit." Dr. Mark Hyman was the host and he interviewed about 30 doctors, pharmacists, and other health professionals. The topic of these interviews was how the body needed healthy fats to heal and function properly. Also, that we need to choose: either a low fat, high carb diet, or a high fat, low carb diet--because a diet high in both fat and carbs was causing a lot of health issues. They went through case studies, personal testimonies, and other resources to show how a low carb, higher fat diet was healing people of various disease.   I then read books written by various presenters, and they too, had the same thing in common: real whole food, getting daily exercise, good sleep, sunlight, and avoiding processed foods.

The second summit that changed my life was "<u>The Diabetes Summit</u>" in 2017. I heard one of the doctors discuss that we were testing only the side effects of diabetes to manage it (A1C & blood glucose) and not getting to the root cause of the illness. At this time, there is no way to test the actual cause. ***Wait . . . what did he just say???*** High blood sugar numbers were the side effect, but not the actual illness. They also said it could be reversed as if I had never had the disease. I had never heard this before, and it led to lots of questions for Dr. Mel, and lots of research papers and books to read. This changed my whole outlook on autoimmune dis-ease. I set out to be diabetes free by the end of 2017, and succeeded.

There are many summits out there, and I have listed a few in the back of this book. The nice thing is that you can pick and choose what speakers you want to hear from. Most are free, and many have gifts for attending in the form of free ebooks or online classes.

7th piece of the puzzle - The <u>Inform Program</u> and support group. It included a clinically studied nutrition plan and guided support group. There was a weekly discussion topic where we were able to engage with others going through a similar journey. This program is laid out so that the participants can be successful as they go from a SAD diet (Standard American Diet) to a more healing way of life.

All of these programs have worked together for my benefit. Some were a part of my life for a short time; some will be with me for the rest of my life. Even the medical doctors have a place in my care. They are great for crisis care (like an injury), and can monitor your health while you make lifestyle changes. Where they fail is chronic dis-ease. The only way they deal with it is symptom management, and the medicines they use have horrible, even life threatening side effects. They do not treat or even address the cause.

Several programs had nutrition as a part of their program. They are all well researched, based on good science, with the goal of healing your body from dis-ease. They agree on the essentials, focusing on eating whole, real foods: eaten as close to the way God made them as possible, getting exercise, good sleep, sunlight, and avoiding processed foods.

In 2017 I lost 70 pounds for a total of 90 pounds. SUCCESS happened when all the pieces of the puzzle came together. I am betting there still pieces to come, but I am enjoying how it is all coming together for me to become the best me that I can be.

It can be summed up with "I shall do my part by eating whole real foods, getting daily exercise, and leave the results up to Him."

Spine alignment, returned to close to normal bends and alignment. In 2014 x-rays showed my spine was missing its 45 degree curves, and the part that was supposed to be straight had an S shaped curve (scoliosis) in it. 2017 x-rays showed my spine to be straight, and only my 45 degree curve on my neck still needs some work.

Asthma: reversed (actually caused by gluten intolerance).

Bronchitis - stopped having it 3 to 5 times a year.

Immune system strengthened, I no longer catch every cold going around.

Seasonal allergies, went from severe to very rarely affected by them

Non-alcoholic fatty liver disease - reversed.

Gall bladder - healed without surgery.

Malnutrition - healed.

My natural hair color returned from almost 70 percent grey.

Have more energy than I had as an athletic teenager.

Diabetes - reversed/cured (moved to a historical diagnosis in my medical record).

Brain fog - gone, I have great mental clarity and function now.

High blood pressure - gone.

Acid reflux/indigestion - gone.

Frequent migraines and headaches - extremely rare now.

Depression - mood has stabilized without medicine.

Hormonal mood swings - stable.

Hormonal hot flashes - gone.

Leaky gut - healed.

Adrenal fatigue - healed.

Sharp stabbing pain when I ate - gone.

Sleeping without having to use drugs.

Went from 11 prescriptions to 1 (thyroid.)

All blood work is now in the normal healthy range.

Started out in a very tight size 28 (refused to buy a larger size) to a comfortable size 16/18. And my shoe size went from a 11W to a 10, in most styles.

What I want you to understand from this story is that while I believe in the power of chiropractic care, and even encourage you to find a good DC in your area. It can only do so much: what you eat, and--more importantly--what you *do not* eat can be the difference between being sick and tired all the time and having so much energy the kids are begging you to slow down (yes, this happened to me.)

Currently I still have a low functioning thyroid, sleep apnea and insulin resistance/metabolic syndrome. They will take time to reverse and so staying the course on a whole food, low carb diet is important.

Also I am dealing with degenerative disc disease in my lower back starting at the waist and down into the buttocks area. After several procedures, physical therapy, and medicines, I have reached the limit of what can be done with moderate success.

The MDs have told me that "it will get worse," and eventually I "will need surgery." but to "stay as active as possible with core muscle strengthening exercises such as yoga, water aerobics, gardening, etc," to delay the surgery. If I do not keep active the discs will only degenerate faster because these core muscles support the spine. I get daily exercise as well as housework and gardening along with frequent rest periods. This disease affects how I plan my whole day, and what I can do with my family.

At this time, the surgery they are discussing has a projected success of only 50/50. It would remove a large portion (25%) of a vertebra to try to relieve the pinched nerves. It does nothing to address the other issues associated with this disease. Now that is a 50% chance of improving the pain only for a few years, after which it gets worse (understand that: they didn't project that it "might" get worse; they promised me that it WILL). Their only other scenario was a 50% chance that I would wake up and be immediately much worse. Let's also not forget the normal risks involved in any surgery. NO THANK YOU.

The medicine they had given me barely helped with the pain. What it did a marvelous job at was making me sleepy, unable to think clearly, drive a car, or return to work. Let's not forget that it was a controlled substance that leads to drug addiction. I have had greater relief from Hemp CBD oil, curcumin, and other herbs, all with the approval of the MD, ND and DC. The herbal supplements help nourish the bones and cartilage as well as helping the pain and inflammation. My goal is to keep it from getting worse and if possible heal completely. Again, the results are up to God.

I got a shock when I asked the doctor why I had this disease at 50 years of age. My grandmother was able to be active well into her 80's. Her response was disturbing. She said, "It's all the processed foods we are eating, and those over the counter pain medications are changing how our brain feels pain. The damage is now done and there is nothing you can do to fix it."

Being unable to work at 50 was not the retirement plan I had in mind. Nutrition matters! Is this reversable? I am not sure. But the alternative is to do nothing, and see the illness progress . . . possibly ending up in a wheelchair, on medications that will leave me unable to do the simplest of tasks.

I am going to choose the path that offers the hope of a full recovery. Either way I will still praise God.

Nutritional Tidbits

Nutritional tidbits, or random truths I have learned over the last 4 years. Feel free to disagree and do your own research. You can never go wrong when you are a seeker of truth whether it be nutrition or daily time with God.

Hippocrates said many, many years ago "Let food be thy medicine and medicine be thy food." In our vast knowledge we have forgotten that the quality and type of food MATTERS. I have heard several functional medicine talks that discuss that chronic disease was almost unheard of until the early 1900's. Children are now coming down with adult onset diseases and it is only expected to get worse.

Eating real whole foods is cheaper than most people think for many reasons.
1. Your body is being nourished so it is not asking for food all the time. (cravings)
2. Since you are satisfied, you will not need to do all the snacking that is done on the SAD diet.
3. Junk food is expensive . . . especially from a vending machine. It also puts you on a insulin high then crash cycle where you are headed back to the vending machine for another pick-me-up. Currently, are you adding the trips to the vending machine to your food budget?
4. You produce much less trash by eating a majority of foods that do not need a box. It also reduces your carbon footprint.
5. You will find yourself able to use a small grocery cart instead of filling up a large one.

The root word "pharma" literally means poison. Ponder that one for a while.

Doctors, even though they spend many years in school are not taught the relationship between food and health. They are lucky if they get more than **one** 60 to 90 minute class on nutrition. Most doctors who have studied nutrition have done so because of their own health issues, and end up switching to another medical model such as chiropractic, functional, or naturopathic medicine.

I use the word dis-ease, on purpose, because we miss that "disease" is the opposite of "ease", or the natural state our bodies were designed to be in. We have to figure out what is causing this disruption in our ease and be willing to make required changes. The choice is between taking a medicine to help with the side effects of the dis-ease or to fix the dis-ease with lifestyle changes. Our bodies were designed to heal and are wonderfully made.

Autoimmune dis-ease is generally caused by what we put into or on our bodies or environment. While that may sound discouraging it is also GREAT NEWS because if we can give ourselves these dis-eases then we can also reverse them. Maybe not totally, but any improvement means less medicine, less pain, less money spent on a medical care, and a better quality of life. What is the other option? Do not make any lifestyle changes, then keep getting sicker, adding more diagnoses, which means more medicine, more pain, more side effects, and more whining about your quality of life.

As for me, I am getting up, pulling on my overalls, and getting to work. God has more planned for me than dis-ease.

Overalls, you asked? Well, Thomas Edison said it best: "Opportunity is missed by most people, because it is dressed in overalls, and looks like work." Well, my overalls are on, and going to stay on. Care to join me?

Yes, Jesus ate bread. But the bread of the Bible was made of many different ingredients: lentils, barley, oats, spelt, dates, etc. They also used many varieties of wheat. As a matter of fact, the only thing the Bible era wheat has in common with what we eat now, is the name. Today's wheat has been genetically modified to increase the yield per acre, then it is highly processed to increase the shelf life. Our bodies were never designed to eat this "wheat." There are still several types of heritage wheat available, but they are hard to find and expensive.

See the bread recipe in Ezekiel 4:9. You can now find Ezekiel Bread (it uses sprouted grains) in the freezer section of many health food stores. I can eat this bread without any stomach discomfort, even though I am gluten intolerant.

The word *essential* when used to discuss nutrition means our bodies can not make it, so we have to get it from our food. There are essential amino acids (protein) and essential fatty acids (fats), but there are no essential carbs (glucose). When our bodies need glucose it can make it from our fat stores and/or protein. We have to consume healthy, good quality proteins and fats. Being on the SAD low fat diet is directly related to my current back issues. Since I was not getting good fats, I was unable to absorb the fat soluble nutrients and minerals that the bones and cartilage needed to be healthy.

Low blood sugar issues are a sign your body is unable to use its own stored fat as a fuel source. That is why people who have low blood sugar spells will often become type 2 diabetic no matter their weight.

Salt and other electrolytes are essential. We get too much sodium from processed foods, but when eating real food we have to add it to the recipes. Check with your doctor for the amount you should be consuming daily, measure it out, and use throughout the day.   Also, like everything else, the source matters: choose real sea salt.

The Keto diet I had to get my carbs lower for a period of time to heal my diabetes. Real Keto has been around for over 150 years. It was originally called the Banting Diet, and was first published in 1863. Some parts of the world still call it Banting. Keto should include real whole food just like this program; the difference is you chose veggies that are lower in carbs, about 20 to 30 grams a day. And the only allowed fruit is berries. It tends to be a little higher fat. But be warned, just like every other diet craze going around, there are people just trying to get rich off of the latest fad. Yes, the quality of ingredients matter for this diet as well. And don't add fat just to add fat.

You can not exercise or supplement your way out of a bad diet. Food choices are 80% of the lifestyle changes you have to make for either weight loss or health gains.

We were designed to move. In July 2017, I was in such severe pain that for weeks I could not get out of bed without help. My muscles atrophied. I still haven't gotten my muscle tone back fully; it has been hard and painful to rebuild the muscle.

My grandmother and several aunts stayed active until well into their 80s, living alone and still taking care of themselves and pets. In Joshua 14:8-13, Caleb was 85 years old and he asked for a tough piece of land for his own. He was still strong and wanted to continue working until the Lord took him home.   It is when we stop moving that we get ourselves in trouble.

When you hear of a study saying some food or food-like substance is either good or bad, go read the study, but more importantly, see who paid for it. All too often, the results favor those who paid for it, no matter what the data shows. There is some good research being done . . . but far too much of it is cherry picked to meet a preset goal of the buyer. They will throw out all data that disagrees with the end results they want. This may mean as much as 90 percent of the data. That is how we got the low fat craze that has so many fat and sick, me included. And if they are advertising study results in TV/magazine ads that is a serious red flag that you need to read the study and see who paid for it.

If your food has to have catchy ads, cartoons, jingles, or fancy, colorful packaging . . . then it is probably something you should avoid.   The more health claims on the front, the more . . . well, you get the idea. If the product is good for you, they do not have to convince you to buy it. A red ripe strawberry or juicy tomato just begs to be enjoyed. No fanfare is needed.

Our bodies replace every cell in our body, on average, every seven years. Some, like our taste buds, take only 10 to 14 days; others take up to ten years. In seven years, will your body be healthier?

The "everything in moderation approach" has been shown to be scientifically inaccurate. It is designed by advertisers as a salve for conscience so you will continue to eat food that is harmful to the body. There is a huge difference between 100 calories of soda, and a 100 calorie apple. Only one of them has any ability whatsoever to heal the body.

As you go through the 13 week program, you will be amazed at how much better you feel, the mental clarity, and overall energy you will gain. Most people choose to stick with the diet plan and make it a lifestyle change. You may be wondering about birthdays or other special events. Enjoy time with your family or friends, pick and choose where you want to follow the meal plan. Do you want a treat such as Aunt Susie's famous chocolate cake? Plan before you get there! I will often stay on the plan for the meal and drinks, but enjoy a small piece of the dessert. I have enjoyed the meal, and the company, but most importantly I have not put myself on an insulin spike and crash cycle.

CAUTION! If you are having "treat days" several times a week, EVERY week . . . then your gut microbiome will end up right back where it was when you started the program.

When eating out, most restaurants will have a meat and vegetable dish. If you do not see what you want, just ask. For example: Italian restaurants can give you their meat sauce over steamed vegetables instead of pasta. The best advice I ever got was to look up the menu online, and have your food choice already made when you get there. That way you can plan to succeed.

At this time I am enjoying the 90 pounds that I have lost. That is 24% of my total body weight at the start. The diet experts say that if you lose over 10% of your body weight you **will** regain all of that weight and then some. But since I am eating whole, real food, my body is letting go of the weight, then doing internal remodeling. When it is ready, it is letting go of more weight. Most people will call the internal remodeling stage a stall. Not me . . . the scale has not moved in a few months, but I have lost inches, lost fat, gained muscle, and gone down another 2 dress sizes. Total non scale victory.

Keep in mind a pound of fat has 7 miles of blood vessels in it. So with each pound lost your body not only has to not only deal with the fat, but also all of the other tissue that was attached and providing nutrients to the cells. I am not fighting or starving my body to lose the weight; instead, I am feeding my body what it needs. My body is now able to do what it was designed to do.

After listening to many doctors in the summits, my whole view of autoimmune dis-ease has changed. I now see it as the body's way of crying out for help. It is saying "I am trying to keep you alive, but I am sick, so I have had to make a sacrifice of this organ or hormone function to save the rest of you. You now have $\underline{X}$; but I am going to try to hold the line here . . . but PLEASE help me by eating better and/or cleaning up the products you use in your home."

...but as for me and my house, we will serve the Lord. Joshua 24:15 This verse is often hung on the wall as a decoration. I see it as more, as a way to live my life. I will tell you the truth according to the word of God. If you do not want to hear it, then do not ask. I am neither smart enough nor arrogant enough to tell the Creator of the universe He is wrong. Period. My job is to tell you the truth; not to police what you do with that truth.

Health application of this verse. There is truth in good dietary science. By the way, good solid science and the Bible agree. The Bible contains much scientific information. In this journey, He has shown me the healing power of eating real, whole foods. Also that dis-ease is caused by what we are eating, especially the food-like substances. It is up to you whether you make changes in the way that you eat or not. *But OWN your decision.* I have heard so many excuses, many from myself, that without judgement, I can now say that if you are not willing to change your diet, then you give up ALL rights to complain about your health issues. ***"The cause is also the cure."*** (Dr. Mel)

The frequent reactions to being shown to the real healing power of nutrition.
1. I can change . . . *Awesome!* I will make use of this opportunity.
2. Do I really have to change the way I eat? It is just too hard, takes too much time, money, etc.
3. "I eat pretty well" (as they fill their cart with 90% processed food.)
4. This is great information, I am glad I learned it . . . but I wonder if my doctor has a pill that will do the same thing as better food choices.
5. Oh my doctor did not suggest improving my diet, so I must be good. But he/she just added some more medicine, oh yeah, also added another dis-ease to my chart.

Seriously: I eat better now than I ever have, and feel amazing. I spend less money on food, medicine, and medical care. I also spend less time in the kitchen.

During the summits, so many of the natural health professionals have discussed how we were designed by God to be self-healing, it is encouraging to hear them acknowledge God and His amazing design.

Daily time with the Lord is *essential:* in prayer, meditation, and in the Book.

"The journey of a thousand miles starts with a single step" unknown.

Devotions

The Bible is   **B**asic
                       Instructions
                       Before
                       Leaving
                       Earth   (Author unknown)

and since He took the time to write it down for us, we might want to read it at least once.

The Bible is an unchangeable, living Book that can guide us through any situation or trial we find ourselves in. We are blessed to be living in a time when the Bible can be freely found and read. Bible study allows us to see and understand who God is.

Every time I read a passage, I learn something new; not because it is different, but because I am different, and ready for deeper understanding of the Word.

The name of this book is "Will thou be made whole?" I had read and heard this story preached on several occasions but not once did I get that it was a question. When I was finally ready to hear that question, you would have thought there was a giant 10' tall neon sign flashing that question at me. Life changing only begins to describe it.

Along this journey, I was being guided by God to other verses, people, or places I needed. Different passages and stories started showing me that in addition to the normally preached upon applications that they could also be applied to nutrition, and the choices we make in food.

I have structured these devotions to address both my own issues and comments heard from others at Bible studies over the years. There are questions that will take you back to the Word, and meditate as well as having room to write down your thoughts. One common complaint has been having to keep up with a separate notebook for notes. I hope you enjoy the format.

I have also included a weekly reflection page so that you have a place to record your goals, wins and losses. Also remember to celebrate the non scale victories.

Just a random thought. The word "universe" means single spoken word. Ponder that the next time you read the creation story.

1 After this there was a feast of the Jews; and Jesus went up to Jerusalem.

2 Now there is at Jerusalem by the sheep market a pool, which is called in the Hebrew tongue Bethesda, having five porches.

3 In these lay a great multitude of impotent folk, of blind, halt, withered, waiting for the moving of the water.

4 For an angel went down at a certain season into the pool, and troubled the water: whosoever then first after the troubling of the water stepped in was made whole of whatsoever disease he had.

5 And a certain man was there, which had an infirmity thirty and eight years.

6 When Jesus saw him lie, and knew that he had been now a long time in that case, he saith unto him, Wilt thou be made whole?

7 The impotent man answered him, Sir, I have no man, when the water is troubled, to put me into the pool: but while I am coming, another steppeth down before me.

8 Jesus saith unto him, Rise, take up thy bed, and walk.

9 And immediately the man was made whole, and took up his bed, and walked: and on the same day was the sabbath.

10 The Jews therefore said unto him that was cured, It is the sabbath day: it is not lawful for thee to carry thy bed.

11 He answered them, He that made me whole, the same said unto me, Take up thy bed, and walk.

12 Then asked they him, What man is that which said unto thee, Take up thy bed, and walk?

13 And he that was healed wist not who it was: for Jesus had conveyed himself away, a multitude being in that place.

14 Afterward Jesus findeth him in the temple, and said unto him, Behold, thou art made whole: sin no more, lest a worse thing come unto thee.

15 The man departed, and told the Jews that it was Jesus, which had made him whole.
John 5:1-15

Jesus asked the man if he would like to be made whole, we see his response. I think it was a human response . . . since he may not have known who Jesus was, and that He had the power to make him whole.   But you know who Jesus is, and you now have the same question placed before you. How will you answer Him?

____

____

____

____

____

The man had been in this condition for 38 years. It was the only life he knew. Consider the fact that he had to depend on the kindness of others to have all his needs met. Now he was faced with being in control of his own future needs. I imagine he felt both joy and fear in his new situation.

What changes will there be for you? Will there be physical or mental roadblocks that you will have to overcome? How are you going to prepare for them?

____

____

____

____

____

Jesus knew how long the man had been at the well, and the challenges that he faced before He ever approached him. Jesus also knows this is a personal journey, and that none of us have the same issues or challenges.

For me, being made whole is to be free of all medical issues and being at a healthy weight. But also being able to be active and have the energy to take care of my family's needs and wants.

What does being whole look like for you?

____

____

____

____

____

Are there any resources that you need to be made whole?

____

____

____

____

____

Jesus told the man to "*Rise, take up thy bed, and walk.*" What I hear is Jesus saying "I have given you what you need, now get up and get started with the rest of your life."

Where do you want to be one year from now?

____

____

____

____

____

5 years from now?

____

____

____

____

____

Notes and thoughts:

____

____

____

____

____

____

____

____

____

____

____

____

____

____

____

____

____

<u>Weekly Questions</u> This is a great way to look back and celebrate the non scale victories, see how far you've come as well as make some plans for the upcoming week.

What is one change I want to make this week?

____
____
____
____

What if any resources do I need to make this change? (time, money, or help from others)

____
____
____
____

What exercise am I going to plan? Maybe try something new?

____
____
____
____

What wins have I had this week? Non scale victories count just as much as the number on the scale.

____
____
____
____
____
____

What things did not go so well and need to change for next week?

____
____
____
____
____

16 Know ye not that ye are the temple of God, and that the Spirit of God dwelleth in you?
17 If any man defile the temple of God, him shall God destroy; for the temple of God is holy, which temple ye are.
1 Corinthians 3:16-17

As His temple, if we are sick, then we will not be able to focus on the mission that He has for us. What are your health issues holding you back from doing?

____

____

____

____

____

These verses should convict you, being the truth of God. Use it as a learning tool instead of beating yourself up. Too many times we get down on ourselves and just quit. NO! Turn that around and realize you were created by a Loving Father who wants more for you. The Creator of the universe loves you and sent His Son for you. You are worth more than you know.   List some of the blessings He has put in your life.

____

____

____

____

____

You have heard the Words that you as His temple are holy. Does this change the way you feel about junk food, or the excuses we make?

____

____

____

____

Are there any self-sabotage issues that need to be dealt with?

____

____

____

____

____

A temple is a place holy and separate to a purpose. Our bodies are a vessel for our soul, His Holy Spirit. God has a mission for each of us. Everything I have been through has been leading me here: to this place, to this time, to share the healing power of nutrition for His glory.

What is your mission?

____
____
____
____
____

God puts people/opportunities in our path at just the right time. Do you have any self-preparation so that you are ready when He places people or opportunities in your path? Maybe you have some uncluttering to do so that you have room for what He is preparing you for.

____
____
____
____
____

Notes and thoughts:

____
____
____
____
____
____
____
____
____
____
____
____
____
____
____

<u>**Weekly Questions**</u> This is a great way to look back and celebrate the non scale victories, see how far you've come as well as make some plans for the upcoming week.

What is one change I want to make this week?

____
____
____
____

What if any resources do I need to make this change? (time, money, or help from others)

____
____
____
____

What exercise am I going to plan? Maybe try something new?

____
____
____
____

What wins have I had this week? Non scale victories count just as much as the number on the scale.

____
____
____
____
____

What things did not go so well and need to change for next week?

____
____
____
____

3 Behold, we put bits in the horses' mouths, that they may obey us; and we turn about their whole body.

4 Behold also the ships, which though they be so great, and are driven of fierce winds, yet are they turned about with a very small helm, whithersoever the governor listeth.

5 Even so the tongue is a little member, and boasteth great things. Behold, how great a matter a little fire kindleth!

6 And the tongue is a fire, a world of iniquity: so is the tongue among our members, that it defileth the whole body, and setteth on fire the course of nature; and it is set on fire of hell.

7 For every kind of beasts, and of birds, and of serpents, and of things in the sea, is tamed, and hath been tamed of mankind:

8 But the tongue can no man tame; it is an unruly evil, full of deadly poison.

9 Therewith bless we God, even the Father; and therewith curse we men, which are made after the similitude of God.

10 Out of the same mouth proceedeth blessing and cursing. My brethren, these things ought not so to be.

11 Doth a fountain send forth at the same place sweet water and bitter?

12 Can the fig tree, my brethren, bear olive berries? either a vine, figs? so can no fountain both yield salt water and fresh.

James 3:3-12

These verses discuss an unbridled tongue and it is often used to discourage gossiping and idle words. But it could also be used to discuss the food choices we make. In the past, our tongue has helped us decide if something is good and safe to eat. The closer we eat food to the way God made it, the healthier we will be.

But today we have scientists creating the "yum" factor in a lab to confuse the tongue into thinking processed foods are good and safe to eat.

How are you going to change your food choices for yourself and your family?

____

____

____

____

____

____

It says the tongue is also a fire that can corrupt the whole body. I agree. What we eat can either heal the body, or cause dis-ease. Are you ready to take control of your tongue, and feed your body healthy foods that nourish it?

____

____

____

____

____

With our tongues, we can also praise the Lord. What are you thankful for today?

____

____

____

____

____

Any specific prayer requests you need to add to your prayer journal? If you do not have a prayer journal yet, now is a great time to start. It helps you see answered prayers and also to be specific in your prayer requests.

____

____

____

____

____

____

____

____

Notes and thoughts:

____

____

____

____

____

____

____

____

____

____

____

<u>**Weekly Questions**</u> This is a great way to look back and celebrate the non scale victories, see how far you've come as well as make some plans for the upcoming week.

What is one change I want to make this week?

____

____

____

____

What if any resources do I need to make this change? (time, money, or help from others)

____

____

____

____

What exercise am I going to plan? Maybe try something new?

____

____

____

____

What wins have I had this week? Non scale victories count just as much as the number on the scale.

____

____

____

____

____

What things did not go so well and need to change for next week?

____

____

____

____

47 And that servant, which knew his lord's will, and prepared not himself, neither did according to his will, shall be beaten with many stripes.
48 But he that knew not, and did commit things worthy of stripes, shall be beaten with few stripes. For unto whomsoever much is given, of him shall be much required: and to whom men have committed much, of him they will ask the more.
Luke 12:47-48

29 For unto every one that hath shall be given, and he shall have abundance: but from him that hath not shall be taken away even that which he hath.
Matthew 25:29

Both of these texts discuss being a wise steward of whatever talent or opportunity God has given to us. He could have chosen to bring us home right after we accepted Him. However, if you are still here, He has given you time to increase the talents He has given you. How are you using your talents?

____

____

____

____

____

The text says that *whomsoever much is given, of him shall be much required*. What has the Lord given you much of . . . time, money, energy, love, ability, etc.?

____

____

____

____

____

How are you increasing your talents or growing for the Lord?

____

____

____

____

____

____

The verses also discuss a chastisement for not increasing the talents that He has given to you. A good Father disciplines his child. If you need to increase your gifts, what is your goal to start?

For Example: It could be turning off the TV or other media an hour before you go to bed to pray and read your Bible. It could be reading the Bible to your children. This will change as you go through the different seasons in your life.

____
____
____
____
____
____
____

Notes and thoughts:

____
____
____
____
____
____
____
____
____
____
____
____
____
____
____
____
____
____
____
____
____

<u>**Weekly Questions**</u> This is a great way to look back and celebrate the non scale victories, see how far you've come as well as make some plans for the upcoming week.

What is one change I want to make this week?

____

____

____

____

What if any resources do I need to make this change? (time, money, or help from others)

____

____

____

____

What exercise am I going to plan? Maybe try something new?

____

____

____

____

What wins have I had this week? Non scale victories count just as much as the number on the scale.

____

____

____

____

____

What things did not go so well and need to change for next week?

____

____

____

____

____

Week 5

This has been a tough lesson to write for me but I felt led to stay the course. I hope it helps you, if you are dealing with the pain of abuse or neglect. This week's Bible verses discusses a "railer." Well, I had to look that one up to see what it meant when the King James Bible was written.   A railer is a small word with a huge meaning.

RA'ILER, n. One who scoffs, insults, censures or reproaches with opprobrious language. *Noah Webster's American Dictionary of the English Language, 1828 Edition*

Opprobrious synonyms; abusive, contemptuous, damaging, derogatory, disparaging, shaming, insulting, offensive, defamatory, untrue, venomous; scornful, *thesaurus.com*

My railer chose to pass on the abuse they suffered as a child. A child understands the difference between abuse and loving discipline. But my abuser tried to convince me that it was my fault . . . or at very least I just imagined it. At school, church, etc. and with extended family I was encouraged; at home, just the opposite. It was confusing and often a scary way to grow up. They tried to hide the abuse from everyone, but a few years after we moved away, several people admitted to me that they hated seeing the way I was treated, but did not feel it was their place to say or do anything.

I spent too many years confused, hurt, lonely, unsure of myself, wanting the truth to come out, and using food/weight to protect myself. I am glad God sent my husband into my life because he gave me strength I needed and helped me continue to heal through listening, observing, and Bible study. I have found great comfort in Psalm 119:165 *Great peace have they which love thy law: and nothing shall offend them.* God is my Rock and I will stand on His truth.

I would like to say the situation has improved, but it has only gotten worse since I have started following God's protocols. (1 Corinthians 5:11) But they have railed even harder, involving more people, pretending that they are the victims. My behavior has not always been the best; I have no problem being corrected with truth, but fight (often stupidly) when condemned with lies. I fear that it will not be settled on this earth but in heaven with Jesus as the judge.   Luke 8:17 says *For nothing is secret, that shall not be made manifest; neither any thing hid, that shall not be known and come abroad.* Or Proverbs 28:13 *He that covereth his sins shall not prosper: but whoso confesseth and forsaketh them shall have mercy.* If this matter waits on Jesus to mediate an honest conversation then the truth will come out for **all to see . . .** not just those involved.

I felt led to share this glimpse into my personal pain and hope it gives comfort those who need to hear "you are not alone."

32 And be ye kind one to another, tenderhearted, forgiving one another, even as God for Christ's sake hath forgiven you. Ephesians 4:32

14 For if ye forgive men their trespasses, your heavenly Father will also forgive you:
15 But if ye forgive not men their trespasses, neither will your Father forgive your trespasses. Matthew 6:14-15

11 I wrote unto you in an epistle not to company with fornicators:
10 Yet not altogether with the fornicators of this world, or with the covetous, or extortioners, or with idolaters; for then must ye needs go out of the world.
11 But now I have written unto you not to keep company, if any man that is called a brother be a fornicator, or covetous, or an idolater, or a railer, or a drunkard, or an extortioner; with such an one no not to eat. 1 Corinthians 5:9-11

God can only forgive us of our sins when we repent. In VBS it is often called the ABCs of salvation, **a**dmit (repent), **b**elieve and **c**onfess (ask forgiveness). Forgiveness without repentance is man's way . . . or put another way, man says to forgive but not forget. God's way is to have a private conversation, an act of true repentance, and then forgiveness. By forgiveness, He expects us to let it go, and NEVER pick it up again, as if it never happened. See Matthew 18:21-22. If we do not forgive others when they ask, then He clearly says He will not forgive us.

Now there are those that will disagree saying "I can just forgive those who have hurt me" and I thought so, too--at the beginning--because the modern definition of forgiveness in many self help books is *"to let go of the anger."* But I struggled with this as a Bible lesson. When I asked my husband for assistance and he took the Word and showed me where this was wrong. Then God showed me both through His Word and in real life where the modern definition of forgiveness was not His way.

We serve a *just* God and He has created us to desire justice. As long as that injustice has not been dealt with it will be a part of our lives; we may stuff it down, maybe with food, indifference, self-worth issues, etc: it is still a part of us until we get justice.

Look at Joseph. God used him to save 2 nations, he was given a good life. But when facing his brothers, he still wanted justice. Both parties were hurting. It was only after the injustice was addressed that his family was healed. Every incident I found in the Bible involved a minimum of 2 people, the hurter and the hurtee, both needed to deal with the issue, together. There are several example of intercessory prayers for those who have hurt us, the most famous of these can be found in Luke 23:34-35.

Forgiveness with those who have hurt us must wait on a honest conversation and true repentance. Still, it is we who must choose whether or not to hold onto the pain, anger, or resentment associated with their actions. We can give it to God, and allow Him to handle the reconciliation. But we need leave it with Him and not pick it up again. He will deal with it, either on earth or in heaven.

Is there pain or anger that you need to stop holding onto, and give to God to handle? Be specific, give it to God in prayer, heal and move forward.

____

____

____

____

____

____

____

____

____

____

____

____

____

____

____

____

Holding onto pain, anger and resentment can affect our relationship with food and others. It is often seen as a protective barrier; actually, it isolates us from good people and events in our lives. Do you have a healthy relationship with food? Is it nourishment . . . or is it comfort (self-medication)?

____

____

____

____

How do you want to change the way you deal with food or others?

____

____

____

____

Holding onto pain, anger and resentment can also affect our health. There are studies that show that the abuse alone can trigger an autoimmune illnesses. For more information, search Niki Gratrix and ACE Score studies.

Holding onto this pain only hurts us; it does nothing to the person that hurt us. But God has an alternative. In addition to 1 Corinthians 5:11, He also gave us the instruction to pray for them.

27 But I say unto you which hear, Love your enemies, do good to them which hate you, 28 Bless them that curse you, and pray for them which despitefully use you.
Luke 6:27-28

Add them to your prayer journal and decide how you are going to pray for them. One of mine has been that God will provide an opportunity for a healthy relationship to develop as well as for them to have a closer relationship with God.

What are some things that you can pray for this person/people?

____
____
____
____
____
____
____
____
____

Notes and thoughts:

____
____
____
____
____
____
____
____
____
____
____
____
____
____
____
____

<u>**Weekly Questions**</u> This is a great way to look back and celebrate the non scale victories, see how far you've come as well as make some plans for the upcoming week.

What is one change I want to make this week?

____
____
____
____

What if any resources do I need to make this change? (time, money, or help from others)

____
____
____
____

What exercise am I going to plan? Maybe try something new?

____
____
____
____

What wins have I had this week? Non scale victories count just as much as the number on the scale.

____
____
____
____
____

What things did not go so well and need to change for next week?

____
____
____
____

This is a continuation to last week's lesson.

32 And be ye kind one to another, tenderhearted, forgiving one another, even as God for Christ's sake hath forgiven you. Ephesians 4:32

14 For if ye forgive men their trespasses, your heavenly Father will also forgive you:
15 But if ye forgive not men their trespasses, neither will your Father forgive your trespasses. Matthew 6:14-15

11 I wrote unto you in an epistle not to company with fornicators:
10 Yet not altogether with the fornicators of this world, or with the covetous, or extortioners, or with idolaters; for then must ye needs go out of the world.
11 But now I have written unto you not to keep company, if any man that is called a brother be a fornicator, or covetous, or an idolater, or a railer, or a drunkard, or an extortioner; with such an one no not to eat. 1 Corinthians 5:9-11

15 Moreover if thy brother shall trespass against thee, go and tell him his fault between thee and him alone: if he shall hear thee, thou hast gained thy brother.
16 But if he will not hear thee, then take with thee one or two more, that in the mouth of two or three witnesses every word may be established.
17 And if he shall neglect to hear them, tell it unto the church: but if he neglect to hear the church, let him be unto thee as an heathen man and a publican.
Matthew 18:15-17

Often those that hurt were hurt themselves. Is there anyone you have hurt that you need to make things right with?

____
____
____
____
____
____
____

Also Ephesians 4:32, He tells us to be *kind, tenderhearted, and forgiving one another . .* He will hold us accountable for how we have behave towards others.

____
____
____
____
____

God gave us the Bible as our Guide. In it, He discusses how to handle railers. Matthew 18:15-17 discusses how we are to handle disagreements, and if unsuccessful then we are to not keep company with, or even have a meal with them. 1 Corinthians 5:11
Why do you think that God gave us this instruction?

____

____

____

____

____

Notice also that Matthew tell us that these matters are to be handled privately. How much more pain is caused when private business is told to anybody or everybody that will listen? Today it is even made worse with social media; with a few keystrokes you can *forever* hurt or be hurt by what is said.

Have you been hurt by private matters being made public, and does this change how you will handle conflict in the future?

____

____

____

____

____

Notes and thoughts:

____

____

____

____

____

____

____

____

____

____

____

____

____

____

____

<u>**Weekly Questions**</u> This is a great way to look back and celebrate the non scale victories, see how far you've come as well as make some plans for the upcoming week.

What is one change I want to make this week?

What if any resources do I need to make this change? (time, money, or help from others)

What exercise am I going to plan? Maybe try something new?

What wins have I had this week? Non scale victories count just as much as the number on the scale.

What things did not go so well and need to change for next week?

1 Now concerning spiritual gifts, brethren, I would not have you ignorant.

2 Ye know that ye were Gentiles, carried away unto these dumb idols, even as ye were led.

3 Wherefore I give you to understand, that no man speaking by the Spirit of God calleth Jesus accursed: and that no man can say that Jesus is the Lord, but by the Holy Ghost.

4 Now there are diversities of gifts, but the same Spirit.

5 And there are differences of administrations, but the same Lord.

6 And there are diversities of operations, but it is the same God which worketh all in all.

7 But the manifestation of the Spirit is given to every man to profit withal.

8 For to one is given by the Spirit the word of wisdom; to another the word of knowledge by the same Spirit;

9 To another faith by the same Spirit; to another the gifts of healing by the same Spirit;

10 To another the working of miracles; to another prophecy; to another discerning of spirits; to another divers kinds of tongues; to another the interpretation of tongues:

11 But all these worketh that one and the selfsame Spirit, dividing to every man severally as he will.

12 For as the body is one, and hath many members, and all the members of that one body, being many, are one body: so also is Christ.

13 For by one Spirit are we all baptized into one body, whether we be Jews or Gentiles, whether we be bond or free; and have been all made to drink into one Spirit.

14 For the body is not one member, but many.

15 If the foot shall say, Because I am not the hand, I am not of the body; is it therefore not of the body?

16 And if the ear shall say, Because I am not the eye, I am not of the body; is it therefore not of the body?

17 If the whole body were an eye, where were the hearing? If the whole were hearing, where were the smelling?

18 But now hath God set the members every one of them in the body, as it hath pleased him.

19 And if they were all one member, where were the body?

20 But now are they many members, yet but one body.

21 And the eye cannot say unto the hand, I have no need of thee: nor again the head to the feet, I have no need of you.

22 Nay, much more those members of the body, which seem to be more feeble, are necessary:

23 And those members of the body, which we think to be less honourable, upon these we bestow more abundant honour; and our uncomely parts have more abundant comeliness.

24 For our comely parts have no need: but God hath tempered the body together, having given more abundant honour to that part which lacked:

25 That there should be no schism in the body; but that the members should have the same care one for another.

26 And whether one member suffer, all the members suffer with it; or one member be honoured, all the members rejoice with it.
27 Now ye are the body of Christ, and members in particular.
28 And God hath set some in the church, first apostles, secondarily prophets, thirdly teachers, after that miracles, then gifts of healings, helps, governments, diversities of tongues.
29 Are all apostles? are all prophets? are all teachers? are all workers of miracles?
30 Have all the gifts of healing? do all speak with tongues? do all interpret?
31 But covet earnestly the best gifts: and yet shew I unto you a more excellent way.
1 Corinthians 12

Gifts of the spirit is a fun topic. My primary gifts are giving and teaching . . . even though I am an introvert, and prefer to work behind the scenes. Even so, He has used me to teach children in preschool, Sunday school, childrens' church, and in very practical but technical trainings in my last job as a civil CAD designer.

Over the last four years I felt Him guiding me, but not the destination. That changed about a year ago, when He provided the opportunity for me to become a certified health coach. In this book, you can see the experience He has given me by using nutrition to reverse many illnesses, and being able to lose 90 pounds. But I still get insecure because I still need to lose another 75 pounds of fat. Let's face it, people are judged more on their appearance than for their experience. He has a reason for putting me in this position while I still have weight to lose, and maybe He will choose to show me why, but until then I will follow where He leads.

As you read through Paul's letter, we are shown that we each make up a valuable part of the body, and that all parts make up the whole. All gifts are important: some teach, some lead, some clean, some build, some heal, etc. What spiritual gifts has God given to you?

____

____

____

____

____

How are you using your gifts for His glory?

____

____

____

____

____

Do you feel him preparing you for a future opportunity, even if you have no idea what it is yet?

____

____

____

____

____

In our society, we often place people on different tiers of importance. But God teaches that each is just as valuable as another in the body of Christ.   For example, the trash collector is just as important as the mayor in the running of a nice, clean, thriving city. Each has a job to do that complements the other, even if everyone only knows the mayor's name.

Think about your role at work, with your family, or at church. How do your gifts strengthen or complement the gifts of others?

____

____

____

____

____

Notes and thoughts:

____

____

____

____

____

____

____

____

____

____

____

____

____

____

<u>**Weekly Questions**</u> This is a great way to look back and celebrate the non scale victories, see how far you've come as well as make some plans for the upcoming week.

What is one change I want to make this week?

____

____

____

____

What if any resources do I need to make this change? (time, money, or help from others)

____

____

____

____

What exercise am I going to plan? Maybe try something new?

____

____

____

____

What wins have I had this week? Non scale victories count just as much as the number on the scale.

____

____

____

____

____

What things did not go so well and need to change for next week?

____

____

____

____

____

5 And the king appointed them a daily provision of the king's meat, and of the wine which he drank: so nourishing them three years, that at the end thereof they might stand before the king.

6 Now among these were of the children of Judah, Daniel, Hananiah, Mishael, and Azariah:

7 Unto whom the prince of the eunuchs gave names: for he gave unto Daniel the name of Belteshazzar; and to Hananiah, of Shadrach; and to Mishael, of Meshach; and to Azariah, of Abed-nego.

8 But Daniel purposed in his heart that he would not defile himself with the portion of the king's meat, nor with the wine which he drank: therefore he requested of the prince of the eunuchs that he might not defile himself.

9 Now God had brought Daniel into favour and tender love with the prince of the eunuchs.

10 And the prince of the eunuchs said unto Daniel, I fear my lord the king, who hath appointed your meat and your drink: for why should he see your faces worse liking than the children which are of your sort? then shall ye make me endanger my head to the king.

11 Then said Daniel to Melzar, whom the prince of the eunuchs had set over Daniel, Hananiah, Mishael, and Azariah,

12 Prove thy servants, I beseech thee, ten days; and let them give us pulse to eat, and water to drink.

13 Then let our countenances be looked upon before thee, and the countenance of the children that eat of the portion of the king's meat: and as thou seest, deal with thy servants.

14 So he consented to them in this matter, and proved them ten days.

15 And at the end of ten days their countenances appeared fairer and fatter in flesh than all the children which did eat the portion of the king's meat.

16 Thus Melzar took away the portion of their meat, and the wine that they should drink; and gave them pulse.

17 As for these four children, God gave them knowledge and skill in all learning and wisdom: and Daniel had understanding in all visions and dreams.

Daniel 1:5-17

Daniel and his friends would have grown up following the dietary laws but when they chose in their hearts to keep them while in captivity, God provided a way. These young men (presumably teenagers but exact age unknown) asked to eat pulse or food grown from a seed. At the end of 10 days they looked better than the other captives and therefore were allowed to continue. Why do you think they were much healthier?

____

____

____

____

The king's meat and wine would have been very rich and more than likely much different from the types of foods the young men were used to eating. Physically, how do you think it affected the young men that choose to eat it?

____

____

____

____

____

How did eating processed food affect you before you started this program? After?

____

____

____

____

____

Because Daniel and his friends choose to follow His dietary rules, God gave them knowledge, skill in all learning and wisdom: and Daniel had understanding in all visions and dreams. They were rewarded for following God's way. How can you apply this to your life?

____

____

____

____

____

When choosing what food to purchase ask yourself; ask "is this food as close to the way God made it as possible?" Why do you need to ask this question?

____

____

____

____

Notes and thoughts:

____

____

____

____

____

There are several books called <u>The Daniel Fast,</u> the best one is by Susan Gregory where she has daily Bible lessons as well as following the dietary restrictions. I did this several years ago and would recommend it as a way to get closer to the Lord.

<u>**Weekly Questions**</u> This is a great way to look back and celebrate the non scale victories, see how far you've come as well as make some plans for the upcoming week.

What is one change I want to make this week?

____
____
____
____

What if any resources do I need to make this change? (time, money, or help from others)

____
____
____
____

What exercise am I going to plan? Maybe try something new?

____
____
____
____

What wins have I had this week? Non scale victories count just as much as the number on the scale.

____
____
____
____
____

What things did not go so well and need to change for next week?

____
____
____
____

1 I beseech you therefore, brethren, by the mercies of God, that ye present your bodies a living sacrifice, holy, acceptable unto God, which is your reasonable service.
2 And be not conformed to this world: but be ye transformed by the renewing of your mind, that ye may prove what is that good, and acceptable, and perfect, will of God.
Romans 12:1-2

Our bodies are "*a living sacrifice, holy, acceptable unto God, which is your reasonable service.*" Jesus paid for our sins on the cross so that we could be a living sacrifice for Him. His sacrifice made us holy. The more we move towards serving the Lord, His way, not ours the happier and more fulfilled our lives become. How has your life changed as you serve Him?

____
____
____
____
____

"*be not conformed to this world:*" We walk into any grocery store and the shelves are filled with treats and goodies that the world says is good and easy. How does your food choices affect our ability to serve Him?

____
____
____
____
____

The more I look at food choices as a way to be obedient and say, yes Lord, Your will, not mine: the easier it is to stay away from foods that keep me too sick to serve Him. Do you agree with this statement? Why or why not?

____
____
____
____
____

God does not take away our freewill to make bad choices; but he definitely uses the result of those choices to teach and rebuke us.   Our dis-ease can be used to teach us about His design. His gift of creating a self-healing body is amazing; but in order to fully use this gift we must eat the good foods He also provided.
Not everyone takes advantage of this gift; are you?

____
____
____
____
____

What life choices has God used to teach or rebuke you?

____
____
____
____
____

"be ye transformed by the renewing of your mind, that ye may prove what is that good, and acceptable, and perfect, will of God." He gives us opportunities to renew our minds (lives) so that we can be in His perfect will. How has He used these nutrition classes to renew you for His will?

____
____
____
____
____

Notes and thoughts:

____
____
____
____
____
____
____
____
____

<u>**Weekly Questions**</u> This is a great way to look back and celebrate the non scale victories, see how far you've come as well as make some plans for the upcoming week.

What is one change I want to make this week?

____
____
____
____

What if any resources do I need to make this change? (time, money, or help from others)

____
____
____
____

What exercise am I going to plan? Maybe try something new?

____
____
____
____

What wins have I had this week? Non scale victories count just as much as the number on the scale.

____
____
____
____
____

What things did not go so well and need to change for next week?

____
____
____
____

16 Ye shall know them by their fruits. Do men gather grapes of thorns, or figs of thistles?
17 Even so every good tree bringeth forth good fruit; but a corrupt tree bringeth forth evil fruit.
18 A good tree cannot bring forth evil fruit, neither can a corrupt tree bring forth good fruit.
19 Every tree that bringeth not forth good fruit is hewn down, and cast into the fire.
20 Wherefore by their fruits ye shall know them.
Matthew 7:16-20

22 But the fruit of the Spirit is love, joy, peace, longsuffering, gentleness, goodness, faith,
23 Meekness, temperance: against such there is no law.
Galatians 5:22-23

As the sanctified of Christ, we are set apart from the world to do the work of the Lord. Twice in Matthew 7:16-20 He clearly states that we will be known by our fruit and also tells us how we will recognize good fruit.

Then in Galatians 5:22-23 He discusses what the fruit of the Spirit is. Take some time and search yourself on how you are applying each of these fruits in your life. Do others know you by these fruits?

Over the years words have changed meaning so I have provided definitions of some words in the year 1611 from the website av1611.com. Shown in parentheses.

Love ____

____

____

____

Joy ____

____

____

____

Peace (In a general sense, a state of quiet or tranquillity; freedom from disturbance or agitation; applicable to society, to individuals, or to the temper of the mind.)

____

____

____

____

Longsuffering (Bearing injuries or provocation for a long time; patient; not easily provoked.)

____

____

____

____

Gentleness (Softness of manners; mildness of temper; sweetness of disposition; meekness)

____

____

____

____

Goodness

____

____

____

____

Faith

____

____

____

____

Meekness (Softness of temper; mildness; gentleness; forbearance under injuries and provocations)

____

____

____

____

Temperance (1. Moderation; particularly, habitual moderation in regard to the indulgence of the natural appetites and passions; restrained or moderate indulgence; as temperance in eating and drinking; temperance in the indulgence of joy or mirth. Temperance in eating and drinking is opposed to gluttony and drunkenness, and in other indulgences, to excess.
2. Patience; calmness; sedateness; moderation of passion.)

____

____

____

____

<u>**Weekly Questions**</u> This is a great way to look back and celebrate the non scale victories, see how far you've come as well as make some plans for the upcoming week.

What is one change I want to make this week?

____
____
____
____

What if any resources do I need to make this change? (time, money, or help from others)

____
____
____
____

What exercise am I going to plan? Maybe try something new?

____
____
____

What wins have I had this week? Non scale victories count just as much as the number on the scale.

____
____
____
____
____

What things did not go so well and need to change for next week?

____
____
____
____

46 And they came to Jericho: and as he went out of Jericho with his disciples and a great number of people, blind Bartimaeus, the son of Timaeus, sat by the highway side begging.
47 And when he heard that it was Jesus of Nazareth, he began to cry out, and say, Jesus, thou Son of David, have mercy on me.
48 And many charged him that he should hold his peace: but he cried the more a great deal, Thou Son of David, have mercy on me.
49 And Jesus stood still, and commanded him to be called. And they call the blind man, saying unto him, Be of good comfort, rise; he calleth thee.
50 And he, casting away his garment, rose, and came to Jesus.
51 And Jesus answered and said unto him, What wilt thou that I should do unto thee? The blind man said unto him, Lord, that I might receive my sight.
52 And Jesus said unto him, Go thy way; thy faith hath made thee whole. And immediately he received his sight, and followed Jesus in the way.
Mark 10:46-52

The Bible records many healings done by Jesus in His earthly ministry. As you read the story of Bartimaeus, notice the difference in his healing and the man at Bethesda pool (John 5).   Bartimaeus knew Jesus could heal him and even though others were trying to silence him: he cried out to Jesus even louder.

Others in our lives try to derail us when we make changes to help ourselves; or to even follow what the Bible/Jesus guides us to do.   For the most part, I do not think that they are trying to hurt us with comments like; Oh, just one bagel will not be too bad, you're allowed a cheat once in a while; seriously, a cheat is shortcut that gets you to a goal faster not push you farther away from your health goals.

I think one of the main reasons that others try to discourage us from a good, healthy lifestyle: is that it shows them that they need to make changes in their own life. Do you have anyone in your life that is trying to derail your progress? Write down some ways you can respond to them in the future.

____

____

____

____

"And Jesus stood still, and commanded him to be called." WOW, our Lord and Savior took the time to stop and help just one man when many wanted His time. Even today, God is available to us through prayer. Include your health goals to your prayer journal.

____

____

____

____

And he, casting away his garment, rose, and came to Jesus. Bartimaeus cast away his beggar's garment, he did not hold onto it because he had faith that he would not need it anymore. Then . . . he went to Jesus.

What are you holding onto, maybe it's your "fat clothes" just in case you need them again. This journey for me was different because it was guided by God. As I shrunk out of my clothes they were bagged up and given away. No safety net . . . it was an act of faith that He was in control and had shown me the way to leave it behind me, for good.

In faith . . . what do you need to let go of?

____

____

____

____

"thy faith hath made thee whole." There is that word whole again, Jesus desires to make us all whole if desire it and do what He asks. Today it is rare for a miracle to just happen in the blink of an eye, but He has given you a self-healing body that just needs to be fed the right nutrients. Are you doing what you need to be made whole?

____

____

____

____

Any changes that you need to make to your lifestyle to be make whole?

____

____

____

____

____

____

____

____

Notes and thoughts:

____

____

____

____

____

____

____

____

<u>**Weekly Questions**</u> This is a great way to look back and celebrate the non scale victories, see how far you've come as well as make some plans for the upcoming week.

What is one change I want to make this week?

____

____

____

____

What if any resources do I need to make this change? (time, money, or help from others)

____

____

____

____

What exercise am I going to plan? Maybe try something new?

____

____

____

____

What wins have I had this week? Non scale victories count just as much as the number on the scale.

____

____

____

____

____

What things did not go so well and need to change for next week?

____

____

____

____

____

7 And lest I should be exalted above measure through the abundance of the revelations, there was given to me a thorn in the flesh, the messenger of Satan to buffet me, lest I should be exalted above measure.
8 For this thing I besought the Lord thrice, that it might depart from me.
9 And he said unto me, My grace is sufficient for thee: for my strength is made perfect in weakness. Most gladly therefore will I rather glory in my infirmities, that the power of Christ may rest upon me.
10 Therefore I take pleasure in infirmities, in reproaches, in necessities, in persecutions, in distresses for Christ's sake: for when I am weak, then am I strong.
2 Corinthians 12:7-10

God turned the direction of the Apostle Paul life around 180 degrees. He went from punishing Christians to writing a majority of the New Testament. But as you read His Word, you see that he had a thorn that he had prayed to God to take away. God responded *"My grace is sufficient for thee: for my strength is made perfect in weakness."*

Paul needed this thorn for the glory of God. Why do you think this was?

____

____

____

____

Many times throughout my journey I have had to wonder if He was keeping me where I was to teach me to stop focusing on the scale: to focus on Him instead. I needed the lesson that He was enough for a joy filled life. It was only when I shifted my focus to Him that He gave me some of the desires for my health. Along this journey how have you changed your focus?

____

____

____

____

Too often it is only when we are at our weakest, that we often remember to pray. Every day we need to thank the Lord for the blessings in our lives. Add some of the blessings He has given you recently and give thanks.

____

____

____

____

"for when I am weak, then am I strong" God made Paul strong, He did not take his thorn but provided other opportunities and/or people to help Paul accomplish His purpose for Paul's life.

What opportunities or people has God placed in your life to strengthen you?

____

____

____

____

Notes and thoughts:

____

____

____

____

____

____

____

____

____

____

____

____

____

____

____

____

____

____

____

____

____

____

<u>**Weekly Questions**</u> This is a great way to look back and celebrate the non scale victories, see how far you've come as well as make some plans for the upcoming week.

What is one change I want to make this week?

____

____

____

____

What if any resources do I need to make this change? (time, money, or help from others)

____

____

____

____

What exercise am I going to plan? Maybe try something new?

____

____

____

____

What wins have I had this week? Non scale victories count just as much as the number on the scale.

____

____

____

____

____

What things did not go so well and need to change for next week?

____

____

____

____

____

11 For I know the thoughts that I think toward you, saith the LORD, thoughts of peace, and not of evil, to give you an expected end.
Jeremiah 29:11

He thinks about us . . . wanting peace for us. How does this verse make you feel? Does it make you want to spend more time with Him?

____

____

____

____

____

____

____

As you finish these 13 weeks it is now time to look forward and choose the next leg of your journey. If you have followed the meal plan in the program then your gut microbiome should be healthy. Now is the time to listen to your body, eat good food when your hungry and maybe add in some fasting.

Maybe consider <u>The Daniel Fast</u> by Susan Gregory, keeping in mind God has used her to teach about this fast: but her recipes do contain some unhealthy ingredients such as canola oil. Just make healthy substitutions. The fasting and Bible study will help you grow in your walk with the Lord.

Or

Maybe you need to add intermittent fasting to your day or even fast for several days to gain some health benefits such as autophagy. Check out Dr. Fung on either youtube or his books

Or

Maybe stay the course on this program for a while longer to reach your goals.

Or

Maybe your health issues need you to cut down on your carbs and try a ketogenic diet.

No matter which path you choose, continue to eat real, whole foods as close to the way God made them as possible.

Read the Bible, pray and meditate for guidance on the next step of your journey.

Notes and thoughts:

Looking back what have been your favorite successes and accomplishments?

Tips to help you succeed.

When you bring fruits and veggies home clean them and prep them as much as possible for the coming week. This will allow you to only have to cleanup peelers, knives and cutting boards once. For ones that you are using as snacks, go ahead and portion them up.

Buy an already prepared tray of organic veggies and divide them up into portions. Yes this costs a little more but can save you time in preparing and cleanup.

Every night as you cook dinner, also prepare breakfast and lunch for the next day so you can just grab and go as you head out the door.

Buy the best possible ingredients you can afford. Grass fed, wild caught, organic and antibiotic free are the best but start where you can and as you can choose better quality.

Organic frozen vegetables are a great time and money saver. It also cuts down on waste from fresh ones going bad before you can eat them. Since they are blanched as part of the preservation and packaging, the portion size will generally be that of cooked vegetables.

Look for time savers like buying already boiled eggs, rotisserie chicken, cooking once and eating several times, or have a day with your spouse or a friend where you prep meals to place in the freezer for the week or month. It is just as easy to make 4 pans of Italian Casserole as it is to make 1. Then you just have to take it out the day before, let it thaw in the refrigerator and bake when you get home.

An electric pressure cooker or crock pot is a great time saver. And with the pressure cooker you can set the timer and it will stop cooking and keep the food warm until you can get to it. Also makes a great hard boiled egg cooker.

I use coconut oil and butter interchangeably in recipes, it depends on the finished flavor I want that night or what I have on hand.

Grass fed butter has some great nutrients, CLA, Vitamins A, D, E, B12 and K2 and also the fat helps you absorb these nutrients.

The menus are based on the basic meal plan of no grains, or sugar. 6 servings of veggies, 1 serving of fruit, 5 ounces of greens and 3 servings of protein and 2 half portions of protein as snacks. For more information see the Facebook page or email me.

Breakfast: choose one daily, see recipes in next chapter.

Breakfast Shake - I often make it the night before so that it is ready to grab from the refrigerator and go in the morning. Or make a blender full and divide between containers. That way you are only making them every other day.

Omelette or scrambled eggs
Low carb Pancakes or Waffle, weekend breakfast option
1 cup 4% cottage cheese with berries
1 cup 4% plain greek yogurt with berries and or seed granola

Snacks Choose 2 daily, using the serving size guide in module 1, see module 1 for other ideas

Hard boiled egg with serving of vegetables such as celery, cucumber, bell peppers, etc.
½ cup 4% cottage cheese with serving of vegetables
Favorite nuts or seeds
Hummus and vegetables to dip
Cheese cubes and vegetables
Cheese cubes and olives
Plain greek yogurt with a serving of fruit.
½ portion of the breakfast shake

Lunch and Dinner
This meal plan has been designed to make it as easy as possible. Both the meal plan and recipes are for 2 people with 4 servings, one portion to eat for dinner and leftovers to eat for lunch the next day. I have tried to make this cook once and eat 2 or 3 times. Feel free to double the recipe and freeze some portions. Vegetables are shown as a minimum, and your protein requirements will be based on your needs, when quantities are show it is an assumed 4 to 5 ounces per person, adjust as needed to meet your macros.

Seasoning - please add them to your taste whether it be just salt, pepper, garlic or your favorite blends

I have given you 2 weeks worth of pre-planned menus. These might work for me but maybe you want a large salad every day for lunch or like me you are not a fan of salads and put your greens in another way. There are several blank menu forms so that you can customize the menu to your tastes.

Beverages - Drink water either plain or with added fruit or herbal teas

Sweeteners - I use liquid stevia, Swerve, Lakanto or xylitol. All of these are all natural but check for added ingredients. I prefer to use stevia in beverages and use xylitol in baked goods. However, Xylitol is toxic to dogs. I grind all the powdered sweeteners in a spice grinder to improve the texture.

Week 1	Lunch	Dinner
Sunday	Baked boneless chicken (cook double for Mondays salad) 2 servings of favorite vegetables	Hamburger steaks Baked vegetable fries Side salad with dressing
Monday	Chicken Salad Greens with dressing Leftover diced chicken 1 cup vegetables	Italian casserole* Green beans
Tuesday	Leftover Italian casserole Or Shake	Tacos Romaine lettuce leaves for shells 1.25 lb Ground beef with 1 cup onions and 1 cup green peppers (divided) cook in coconut oil Taco seasoning (homemade)* Favorite toppings such as tomatoes, olives, salsa, avocado, and cheddar cheese
Wednesday	Taco salad Greens with salsa for dressing 4 ounces of leftover taco meat Favorite taco toppings 1 cup vegetables	Crock-pot roast with vegetables Cook extra for lunch the next day
Thursday	Side salad with dressing Roast and veggies leftovers	Steak (cook double) Baked sweet potato with butter Vegetable
Friday	Steak salad Greens with dressing Leftover steak 1 cup vegetables	Pizza bake* 1 serving vegetables
Saturday	Grilled or baked kabobs 1 inch cubes of chicken or steak and place on skewers with mushrooms, onions, green peppers, cherry tomatoes, etc.	Leftover night, use this night to finish off any leftovers from the week or Dinner hash

***Recipe in next chapter.**

Week 2	Lunch	Dinner
Sunday	Fish, baked or pan grilled Side salad 2 servings of favorite vegetables	Baked or grilled chicken (cook double) Side salad 2 vegetables
Monday	Chicken Salad Greens with dressing Leftover diced chicken 1 cup vegetables	Designer Soup *
Tuesday	Leftover Designer Soup	Tacos Romaine lettuce leaves for shells 1.25 lb Ground beef with 1 cup onions and 1 cup green peppers (divided) cook in coconut oil Taco seasoning (homemade)* Favorite toppings such as tomatoes, olives, salsa, avocado, and cheddar cheese
Wednesday	Taco salad Greens with salsa for dressing 4 ounces of leftover taco meat Favorite taco toppings 1 cup vegetables	Crockpot beans with ham and vegetables Or Lentil chilli*
Thursday	Side salad with dressing Breakfast shake*	Steak (cook double) Baked sweet potato with butter Vegetable
Friday	Steak salad Greens with dressing Leftover steak 1 cup vegetables	Pizza bake 1 serving vegetables Or Italian casserole
Saturday	Stir fry - diced chicken or steak saute with minced garlic, coconut aminos, sea salt Add in a variety of vegetables such as mushrooms, onions, green peppers, cherry tomatoes, etc.	Leftover night, use this night to finish off any leftovers from the week or Dinner hash

***Recipe in next chapter.**

Week	Lunch	Dinner
Sunday		
Monday		
Tuesday		
Wednesday		
Thursday		
Friday		
Saturday		

Week	Lunch	Dinner
Sunday		
Monday		
Tuesday		
Wednesday		
Thursday		
Friday		
Saturday		

Week	Lunch	Dinner
Sunday		
Monday		
Tuesday		
Wednesday		
Thursday		
Friday		
Saturday		

Week	Lunch	Dinner
Sunday		
Monday		
Tuesday		
Wednesday		
Thursday		
Friday		
Saturday		

Week	Lunch	Dinner
Sunday		
Monday		
Tuesday		
Wednesday		
Thursday		
Friday		
Saturday		

Week	Lunch	Dinner
Sunday	82	
Monday		
Tuesday		
Wednesday		
Thursday		
Friday		
Saturday		

Recipes

<u>Breakfast Shake</u> - Protein: 1; Fat: 2; Greens: 3 ounces; Fruit: 1, optional

For each serving, blend the following:
1 serving shake mix
¼ to ½ of an avocado
3 ounces of frozen greens
1 serving berries, optional
1 TBSP cacao powder (100 mg potassium & 8% of daily magnesium needs)
Stevia drops to taste (optional)
Water and/or coconut milk to the desired thickness

<u>Omelette or scrambled eggs</u> Protein: 1; Fat: 1; Greens: 3 ounces; Vegetables: 1

2 eggs with 3 ounces of spinach, and one serving of vegetables, such as bell peppers or mushrooms, 1 slice of bacon or other meat as a garnish. Use 1 tbsp of butter to keep eggs from sticking and add great flavor. Salt and pepper
Each egg has 7 grams of protein, you can add another egg if you omit the meat.

Tip: This can be made ahead of time as a breakfast bowl. Just make the scrambled eggs separately until almost done and then add to the other ingredients. The eggs will continue to cook when you heat it up. This keeps the eggs from getting rubbery.

<u>Low carb Pancakes or Waffle</u>, weekend breakfast option
Protein: 1; Fat: 2; Fruit: 1; Dairy: 1

Per person, combine in a blender and blend until combined, let sit for 5 minutes and cook as either a pancake or waffle.
2 Tbsp cream cheese
2 Tbsp coconut flour
2 eggs
1 tsp vanilla
1 tsp baking powder
1 tsp cinnamon
2 to 4 drops liquid stevia if desired.

Serve with
2 slices of bacon or sausage or ham. (5 to 8 grams of protein serving size) Or you can replace the meat with an egg.
1 serving of stevia or monk fruit sweetened maple syrup, if desired
1 serving fruit.

Italian casserole - 4 servings (This recipe came from my desire for spaghetti, we prefer it with zucchini but is also tasty with spaghetti squash)
450 Calories - Carbs 10g; Fiber 3g; Fat 30g; Protein 35g

4 cups zucchini squash, chopped (or mix of other veggies, mushrooms, onions, peppers, spaghetti squash etc.)
1 pound italian sausage, browned and drained (can use ground beef and Italian seasoning)
1 jar no sugar added marinara sauce
1 cup shredded mozzarella cheese

Place squash in the bottom of a greased casserole dish, sprinkle with salt and pepper, then layer the sausage, marinara sauce and sprinkle the mozzarella cheese on top. Bake at 350 for 45 minutes until cheese is melted and starting to brown.

Pizza Bake
Slice zucchini squash longways to use as the crust, remove the seeds if desired. Then spoon in no sugar added marinara sauce, pizza toppings such as peppers, mushrooms, italian sausage, pepperoni and mozzarella cheese.

Cook in 350 degree oven until squash is done and cheese is melted, 20 to 30 minutes.

Mild Taco Seasoning or you can find a variety of recipes on Pinterest
For 1 lb of meat

2 tsp. Chili Powder	1 tsp. Cumin
1 tsp. Oregano	1 Tbsp minced Garlic
½ tsp. Onion powder	½ tsp Sea Salt
Dash of pepper	

Dinner Hash - 4 Servings This is a versatile dish that you can customize with about any vegetable or meat that you like. You can even top it with an egg.

4 to 5 cups of vegetables, your choice of sweet potato, beets, carrots, bell peppers, onions, mushrooms, cauliflower, broccoli, summer squash, etc.
Salt and favorite spice blend
Coconut oil to keep from sticking
Stir fry them in a skillet until tender, then add in about a handful of greens per person and cook until they reach desired doneness Divide into 4 bowls/plates and set aside.

Dice up a pound of meat and saute in same skillet with some salt and your favorite spices. Divide between the bowls, sprinkle with fresh herbs if desired and enjoy.
This works well with chicken, steak, shrimp or ground beef

<u>**Designer Soup**</u> - very versatile filling soup Serves 4

In each of 4 bowls place 1 cup grated zucchini (uncooked) and one diced green onion

Choose one meat, saute 4 servings in coconut oil until done, divide between the bowls.

Diced chicken	Ground beef
Diced streak	Shrimp
Diced pork chops	Scallops

Then make the broth and divide between the 4 bowls
Saute 1 cup onions or bell peppers with 2 cloves of minced garlic
Then add 4 cups of chicken bone broth
2 Tbsp coconut aminos
2 Tbsp apple cider vinegar
1 tsp Turmeric
1 tsp Sea Salt
Pepper to taste
Can add red pepper flakes, or ginger, if desired
Can also add a poached egg, if desired.

Lentil Chilli - 4 servings

Can substitute ground beef and/or ground pork, (I normally do a half a pound of each). This recipe is inspired by several different recipes that I have used to adapt my original family recipe.

2 cups dry lentils - cook until tender, drain and set aside

Saute 1 cup diced onions
    1 Tbsp minced garlic
    1 cup bell peppers in 1 Tbsp Coconut oil until tender.

Then return the cooked lentils to the pot with 2-15 ounce cans of organic diced tomatoes and the following seasonings

1 Tbsp Cumin
1 Tbsp Oregano
1 Tbsp Chilli Powder
1 tsp. Turmeric

Simmer for 15 to 20 minutes

<u>Seed Granola - 8 Servings, ½ cup each</u>
Calories 392; Carbs 11g; Fiber 8g; Fat 35g; Protein 12g

1 Tbsp coconut oil, melted, remove from heat and stir in
2 tsp ground cinnamon
20 drops liquid stevia or to taste
1 tsp vanilla

Then pour over the seed mixture and stir until coated
1 cup unsweetened coconut flakes
1 cup pumpkin seeds (unshelled) already roasted and salted
1 cup sunflower seeds, already roasted and salted
1 cup sliced almonds, raw works just fine

Spread evenly on cookie sheet and bake at 250 degrees for 45 minutes, stirring every 15 minutes. Mixture should be dried out and starting to brown. Store in container lined with a paper towel to absorb any excess oil.

<u>Flavored Water</u> It can be hard to enjoy the taste of water, especially if you are used to other beverages. To make it easier you can add fruit and veggie slices into your water, some of the ones that work well are 3 to 4 slices of cucumber, lemons, lime, 1 large sliced strawberry or other sliced berries.

<u>Fizzy Drink</u>
Mineral Water
1 tsp favorite extract
Stevia drops 4 to 6, to taste
Some of my favorite extracts are pineapple, root beer or strawberry.
Pineapple is great with some coconut cream added for a pina colada flavored beverage.

<u>Nut Butter Fat Bomb - 12 servings</u> Use as a small treat
Melt the following over low heat until combined
2 Tbsp Coconut oil
2 Tbsp Butter
4 Tbsp Nut Butter (only ingredients are nuts and salt)
3 Tbsp Cocoa Powder
3 Tbsp Powdered Xylitol or other powdered sweetener, stevia will NOT work

Remove from heat and add
1 Tbsp Vanilla
½ cup unsweetened shredded coconut
Divide into 12 portion cups and sprinkle tops with sea salt
Freeze until firm
Best stored in freezer and then allowed to thaw before eating.

Chocolate Keto Cake - 12 Servings
169 calories - Carbs 2g, 13 g Fat, 8 g protein

Cake
Preheat oven to 350 degrees
12 eggs separated,
Place egg whites in mixing bowl, mix for 1 minute until frothy, add

½ cup egg white powder (optional but makes a firmer cake)
2 tsp cream of tartar
1 tsp. vanilla
1/4 tsp salt
mix on high until stiff peaks form.

In another bowl mix the following together until well blended,
1 cup Swerve or other sweetener of choice
⅓ cup Cacao or cocoa powder
4 egg yolks, (can add more if you want but it will make the cake taste eggy and change the macros)
With the mixer on low add the cocoa mix to the egg whites and stop when just mixed.

Place an oversized sheet of parchment paper in a jelly roll pan or deep cookie sheet. Gently spread batter into prepared pan and bake for 15 to 20 minutes. Let cool completely.

Frosting
1 1/2 heavy whipping cream
1 tsp vanilla
3 Tbsp Sour cream
1/4 cup powdered Swerve
Place in a mixing bowl and whip until soft peaks form
Spread on cooled cake, and roll like a jelly roll or you can cut the cake in thirds and place frosting in between the layers and on top, sprinkle with cacao powder, Enjoy

Variation - Pumpkin roll, add 1/2 can of pumpkin and 2 tsp pumpkin pie spice in place of the cacao. Sprinkle more pumpkin pie spice on top

Basic Custard for leftover egg yolks
4 egg yolks   ¼ cup sweetener
1 cup coconut milk   Flavor, see below
Blend ingredients together in a blender for 2 minutes
Cook over low heat until thick, stirring constantly, chill and enjoy

Lemon, add ¼ cup of lemon juice
or
Chocolate, add 2 Tbsp cocoa powder

Keto bread

Preheat oven to 350 degrees

12 eggs separated,
Place egg whites in mixing bowl, mix for 1 minute until frothy, add
½ cup egg white powder
2 tsp cream of tartar
1 tsp. Salt
mix on high until stiff peaks form.

Then gently add in and stir until just mixed
1 Tbsp combined savory spice blends such as garlic powder, rosemary, oregano, parsley
4 egg yolks, (can add more if you want but it will make it taste eggy)
Optional, 1 cup cheese

Place in oiled bread pan and bake for 40 to 45 minutes and then turn off oven and allow to cool before removing from oven.

Slice and store in the refrigerator for up to a week.
This bread will toast for sandwiches.

For other great recipes you can use Pinterest and search low carb or keto recipes. One word of caution, anyone can post recipes and call them low carb. Check the ingredients before you start.

Helpful Resources

Here are some of the health professionals that I have used throughout my journey. I recommend them for their compassionate knowledge and desire to help you live "your best life."

InVision Family Chiropractic, Dr. Melanie Gartside, D.C.
Maximized Living Franchise
1720 S Walton Blvd Suite 6
Bentonville AR 72712
(479) 464-0834
invisionchiro.com

Belle Journee Spa, Amber Dehn, massage therapist/ owner
1730 SE Moberly Lane #1
Bentonville, AR 72712
(479) 616-1690
bellejourneespa.com

Shipman's Healthy & Whole
1501 S.E. Walton Blvd, Suite 105
Bentonville, AR 72712
(479) 254-9230
They are very knowledgeable on the supplements and products they carry.
They also have 2 Naturopathic Doctors available. I have seen both and would recommend either one.
Jane Manasseri, ND
Marvin Shipman, ND

<u>Various online summits</u>, you can find some past interviews on youtube but most are only available during the yearly summit. I have listed some that appear to be yearly events and the general time they have been held in the past..

The nice thing is that you can pick and choose who you want to listen to because with some of the speakers the information will hit home and others it will be great information for someone else. Once you attend one and you will get emails about others that you might be interested in. You also have the option to purchase the summits so that you can have the information to keep.

There are normally free gifts or ebooks just for attending the summits. Some offer discounts off of eclasses or services. Again you can pick and choose what you need.

Diabetes Summit hosted by Dr. Brian Mowll, held in April
The Fasting Summit hosted by Sam Asher, held in April
Living Pain Free Summit hosted by Sheri Weaver, held in May
Keto 101 Summit held in April
Keto Edge Summit hosted by Dr. David Jockers, held in May
Global Health Summit hosted by Kerry Tepedino, held in June
Candida Summit hosted by Evan Brand held in July
Healthy Gut Summit, held in May
Toxic Home Transformation Summit held in June
Home Medical Summit hosted by Marjory Wildcraft, held in May

Websites or Google searches, Youtube videos that you should explore:
Youtube videos, there are great talk but keep in mind anyone can post on there. Here are just a few resources I use . . .

Lots of medical studies on various topics, most are easy to read and website is user friendly.
www.greenmedinfo.com

Dr. Axe general health information

Dr. Jockers, keto information

Dr. Fung, fasting information

Butter Bob, youtube, he is great for explaining functions of the body on a level that is

easily understood.

Jimmy Moore, youtube, introduction to the keto diet.

Maria Emmerich, solid information for keto and lots of healthy recipes on her website.

Dr. Osborne is helping patients that the medical model has given up on. www.drpeterosborne.com and www.glutenfreesociety.org

And lastly let us not forget to laugh. There are some great Christian comedians to tickle our funny bones on youtube.

Back cover photo by Stephanie Dye

Cheryl McGuire Facebook Page: Will Thou Be Made Whole
Email: bemadewhole23@gmail.com